MEDITARANEAN DIET COOKBOOK FOR TYPE 2 Diabetes

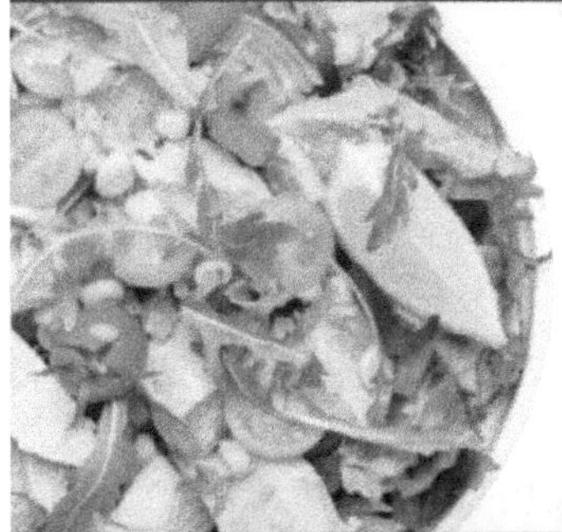

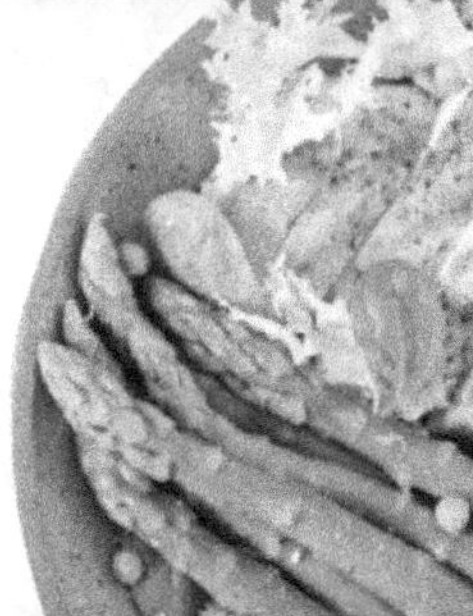

The Ultimate Tasty Low Carb Recipes To Manage And Reverse Type 1 And Type 2 Diabetes

LEONA BUTLER

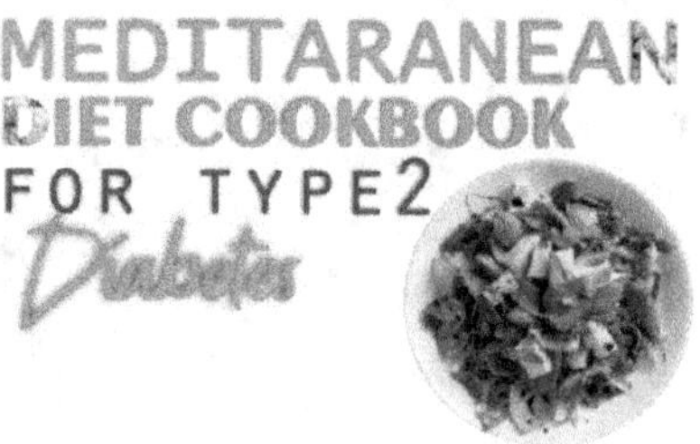
MEDITARANEAN
DIET COOKBOOK
FOR TYPE2
Diabetes

Table of content

39 Nutritious Recipes For Mediterranean Diet Cookbook for Type 2 Diabetes

Introduction

Breakfast Recipes

Lunch Recipes

Dinner Recipes

Snacks Recipes

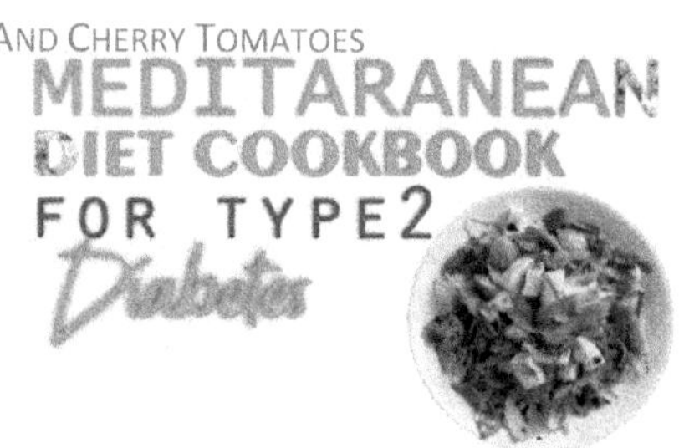

Bonus: 14 Weeks Meal Planner

The Paperback Of This Version Has A Free 14 Weeks Meal Planner

30 Day Meal Plan

Conclusion

Introduction

This Mediterranean diet cookbook for those with type 2 diabetes provides a thorough guide to living a healthy lifestyle. It focuses on the well-known Mediterranean dietary pattern and offers a wide range of delectable meals that adhere to diabetes management standards.

The cookbook promotes blood sugar control and overall well-being by emphasizing nutrient-dense, complete meals high in fiber, antioxidants, and healthy fats. Each cuisine, from vivid salads to savory main courses, is carefully developed to balance flavor, nutritional content, and glycemic impact.

The cookbook also provides helpful hints on portion control, mindful eating, and incorporating physical activity into daily activities. This cookbook serves as a practical companion, encouraging those with type 2 diabetes to experience a delightful and sustainable Mediterranean-inspired culinary adventure while supporting their health goals, thanks to its user-friendly approach and emphasis on healthful ingredients.

Mediterranean diet cookbook for type 2 diabetes

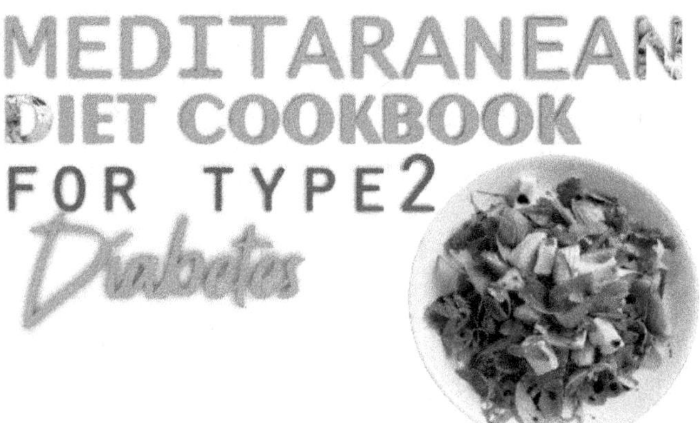

Breakfast Recipes

1. Mediterranean Veggie Omelette

Ingredients:

- 3 large eggs
- 1/4 cup diced red bell pepper
- 1/4 cup diced green bell pepper
- 1/4 cup diced red onion
- 1/4 cup diced tomatoes
- 1/4 cup chopped spinach
- 2 tablespoons feta cheese, crumbled
- 1 tablespoon olive oil Salt and pepper to taste

Preparation:

1. Whisk the eggs in a mixing bowl until completely combined.
2. In a nonstick skillet over medium heat, heat the olive oil.

3. Add red and green bell peppers, red onion, and tomatoes. Sauté for 3-4 minutes until vegetables are tender.

4. Add chopped spinach to the skillet and cook for an additional 1-2 minutes until wilted.

5. Pour the beaten eggs over the sautéed vegetables in the skillet.

6. Sprinkle feta cheese evenly over the eggs.

7. Allow the omelette to cook undisturbed for 2-3 minutes until the edges set.

8. Carefully fold the omelette in half using a spatula.

9. Cook for another 1-2 minutes, or until the center is fully cooked.

10. Season with salt and pepper to taste.

Nutritional Value (approximate):

- Calories: 350
- Protein: 20g

- Fat: 25g

- Carbohydrates: 10g

- Fiber: 3g

Cooking Time: 8-10 minutes

2. Greek Yogurt Parfait

Ingredients:

- 1 cup Greek yogurt

- 1/4 cup granola

- 1/2 cup mixed berries (strawberries, blueberries, raspberries)

- 1 tablespoon honey

- 1 tablespoon chopped nuts (almonds, walnuts)

Preparation:

- In a serving glass or bowl, layer 1/3 cup Greek yogurt at the bottom.

- Add 1 tablespoon granola evenly over the yogurt layer.

- Scatter a handful of mixed berries (about 1/4 cup) on top of the granola.
- Repeat the layering process with another 1/3 cup yogurt, 1 tablespoon granola, and berries.
- Drizzle 1 tablespoon honey over the second layer.
- Finish with the remaining 1/3 cup yogurt, sprinkle the chopped nuts on top.
- Garnish with a few additional berries and a drizzle of honey if desired.

Nutritional Value:

- Calories: Approximately 300-350 kcal
- Protein: Around 15-20g
- Carbohydrates: 30-35g
- Fat: 12-15g
- Fiber: 5-7g

Cooking Time:

Ready to eat in 5-10 minutes.

3. Quinoa Breakfast Bowl

Ingredients:

- cup quinoa
- cups water
- 1 cup almond milk
- 1 tablespoon chia seeds
- 1 tablespoon honey
- 1/2 teaspoon vanilla extract
- 1/2 cup fresh berries (strawberries, blueberries, or raspberries)
- 1/4 cup sliced almonds
- Greek yogurt (optional, for serving)

Preparation:

1. Rinse quinoa under cold water.

2. In a saucepan, combine quinoa and water, bring to a boil, then reduce heat and simmer for 15 minutes until water is absorbed.

3. In a separate saucepan, heat almond milk, chia seeds, honey, and vanilla extract until it thickens slightly.

4. Mix the quinoa with the chia seed mixture.

5. Divide into bowls and top with fresh berries and sliced almonds.

6. Serve with a dollop of Greek yogurt, if desired.

Nutritional Value (per serving):

- Calories: ~400
- Protein: ~12g
- Fiber: ~8g
- Fat: ~15g
- Carbohydrates: ~60g

Cooking Time: 20 minutes.

4. Mediterranean Avocado Toast

Ingredients:

- 2 slices whole-grain bread
- 1 ripe avocado
- 1 tablespoon extra-virgin olive oil
- 1 teaspoon lemon juice
- Salt and pepper to taste
- small tomato, diced
- tablespoons feta cheese, crumbled Fresh basil leaves for garnish

Preparation:

1. Toast the whole-grain bread pieces to taste.
2. Mash the ripe avocado in a bowl while the bread toasts. Add the olive oil, lemon juice, salt, and pepper to taste. Combine thoroughly.
3. Distribute the mashed avocado evenly on the toasted bread slices.

4. Top each slice with diced tomatoes and crumbled feta cheese.

5. Garnish with fresh basil leaves.

6. Serve immediately.

Nutritional Value (per serving):

- Calories: Approximately 350 kcal

- Protein: 9g

- Carbohydrates: 30g

- Fiber: 9g

- Fat: 23g

- Saturated Fat: 5g

- Cholesterol: 10mg

- Sodium: 400mg

Cooking Time:

15 minutes (including toasting time)

Ingredients:

- 2 tbsp olive oil
- onion, finely chopped
- bell peppers, diced
- cloves garlic, minced
- 1 tsp ground cumin
- 1 tsp ground paprika
- 1/2 tsp cayenne pepper (adjust to taste)
- 1 can (28 oz) crushed tomatoes
- Salt and pepper to taste
- 6-8 large eggs
- Fresh parsley, chopped (for garnish)

Preparation:

1. In a large skillet over medium heat, heat the olive oil.
2. Add chopped onions and sauté until translucent.

3. Stir in diced bell peppers and cook until softened.

4. Add minced garlic, ground cumin, paprika, and cayenne pepper. Cook for an additional minute.

5. Pour in crushed tomatoes and season with salt and pepper.

6. Simmer, stirring occasionally, for 10-15 minutes, or until the sauce thickens.

7. Crack the eggs into little wells in the sauce.

8. Cover the skillet and cook until the eggs are done to your liking, approximately 5-7 minutes for runny yolks.

9. Garnish with chopped parsley before serving.

Nutritional Value

- Calories: 250
- Protein: 12g
- Fat: 18g

- Carbohydrates: 15g

- Fiber: 4g

- Sugars: 8g

Cooking Time: 30 minutes

Enjoy your delicious and nutritious shakshuka!

6. Mediterranean Chia Pudding

Ingredients:

- 1/4 cup chia seeds

- 1 cup almond milk

- 1 tablespoon honey

- 1/2 teaspoon vanilla extract

- 1/4 cup chopped dried figs

- 1/4 cup chopped pistachios 1/4 cup pomegranate arils

Preparation:

1. Combine the chia seeds, almond milk, honey, and vanilla essence in a mixing dish.

2. Mix well.

3. Allow the mixture to sit for 15 minutes, stirring occasionally to prevent clumping.

4. Cover the bowl and refrigerate for at least 2 hours or overnight for a thicker consistency.

5. Before serving, stir the pudding to ensure an even texture.

6. Top with chopped dried figs, pistachios, and pomegranate arils.

Nutritional Value (per serving):

- Calories: Approximately 250
- Protein: 7g
- Fat: 15g
- Carbohydrates: 25g

- Fiber: 10g Sugars: 10g

Cooking Time:

Prep Time: 15 minutes

Refrigeration Time: 2 hours or overnight

7. Mediterranean Frittata Muffins:

Ingredients:

- 6 large eggs
- 1/4 cup milk
- 1/2 cup diced bell peppers (red and green)
- 1/2 cup cherry tomatoes, halved
- 1/3 cup crumbled feta cheese
- 1/4 cup black olives, sliced
- 2 tablespoons fresh parsley, chopped
- Salt and pepper to taste Olive oil (for greasing)

Preparation:

19

1. Preheat the oven to 375°F (190°C) and grease a muffin tin with olive oil.

2. Whisk together the eggs and milk in a mixing dish until well mixed..

3. Add diced bell peppers, cherry tomatoes, feta cheese, black olives, and chopped parsley to the egg mixture. Season with salt and pepper.

4. Mix all ingredients until evenly distributed.

5. Fill each muffin cup about 3/4 full with the mixture from the prepared muffin tray.

6. Bake in the preheated oven for 15-20 minutes or until the frittata muffins are set and slightly golden on top.

7. Allow them to cool for a few minutes before removing from the tin.

Nutritional Value

- Calories: ~150

- Protein: ~10g
- Fat: ~11g
- Carbohydrates: ~4g
- Fiber: ~1g
- Sugars: ~2g
- Sodium: ~300mg

Cooking time may also vary, so keep an eye on the muffins to avoid overcooking.

8. Whole Grain Pancakes with Berries

Ingredients:

- 1 cup whole wheat flour
- 1 tablespoon sugar
- 1 teaspoon baking powder
- 1/2 teaspoon baking soda
- 1/4 teaspoon salt
- 1 cup buttermilk

- large egg

- tablespoons melted butter

- 1 teaspoon vanilla extract

- 1 cup mixed berries (blueberries, raspberries, strawberries)

Preparation:

1. In a large bowl, whisk together the whole wheat flour, sugar, baking powder, baking soda, and salt.

2. In a separate bowl, combine the buttermilk, egg, melted butter, and vanilla extract.

3. Stir the wet ingredients into the dry ingredients until just mixed. Make sure not to overmix; a few lumps are fine.

4. Over medium heat, heat a griddle or nonstick skillet. Grease lightly with cooking spray or butter.

5. For each pancake, pour 1/4 cup batter onto the griddle. Top each pancake with a handful of mixed berries.

6. Cook until surface bubbles appear, then flip and cook until the second side is golden brown.

7. Repeat until all the batter is used.

Nutritional Value (per serving):

- Calories: 200

- Protein: 7g

- Fat: 8g

- Carbohydrates: 27g

- Fiber: 4g Sugars: 7g

Cooking Time:

Approximately 3 minutes per side, making a total of around 6-7 minutes for a batch of pancakes.

9. Mediterranean Breakfast Burrito

Ingredients:

- 2 large whole wheat or spinach tortillas

- 4 large eggs

- cup cherry tomatoes, diced

- 1/2 cup cucumber, diced

- 1/4 cup red onion, finely chopped

- 1/4 cup feta cheese, crumbled

- tablespoons black olives, sliced

- 1 tablespoon olive oil

- 1 teaspoon dried oregano Salt and pepper to taste

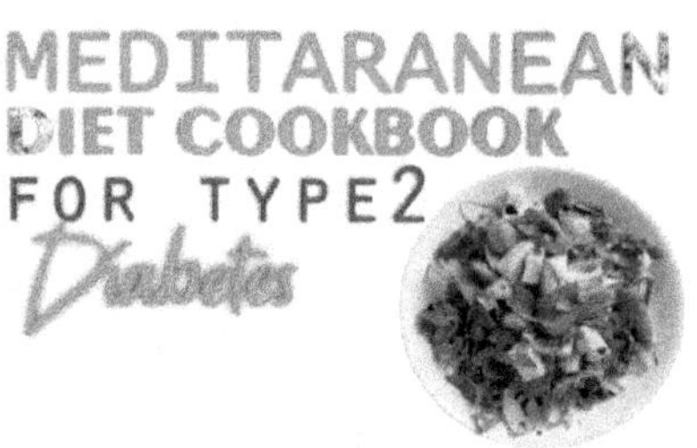

Preparation:

1. In a skillet over medium heat, heat the olive oil.

2. Sauté red onions until softened, then add cherry tomatoes and cook until they release their juices.

3. In a bowl, beat eggs and pour them into the skillet with the vegetables.

4. Scramble the eggs until cooked through, seasoning with salt, pepper, and dried oregano.

5. Warm the tortillas in a separate pan or microwave for about 20 seconds.

6. Assemble the burritos: Divide the scrambled eggs among the tortillas, then top with cucumber, feta cheese, and black olives.

7. Fold the sides of the tortilla over the filling, creating a burrito shape.

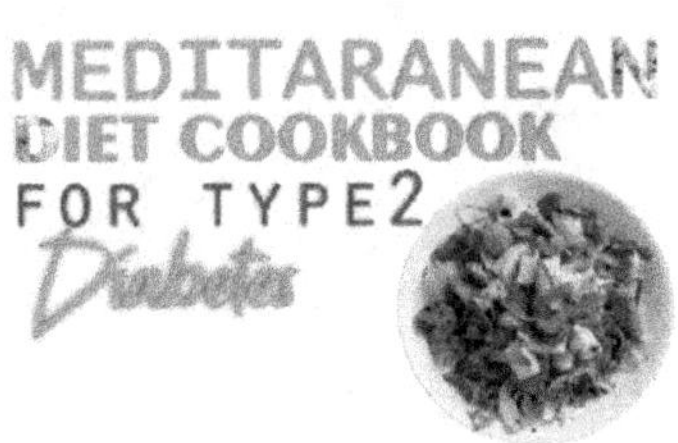

- Nutritional Value (per burrito):

- Calories: approximately 400-450 kcal

- Protein: 20g

- Fat: 25g

- Carbohydrates: 30g

- Fiber: 5g

Cooking Time:

Approximately 15 minutes

10. Smoked Salmon and Avocado Wrap

Ingredients:

- 4 large whole-grain tortillas

- 200g smoked salmon

- 2 ripe avocados, sliced

- cup cherry tomatoes, halved

- 1/2 red onion, thinly sliced

- 1/4 cup fresh dill, chopped
- 1/4 cup cream cheese
- tablespoons lemon juice Salt and pepper to taste

Preparation

1. In a bowl, mix cream cheese with lemon juice, salt, and pepper.
2. Distribute the cream cheese mixture evenly on each tortilla.
3. Layer smoked salmon, avocado slices, cherry tomatoes, red onion, and fresh dill on top of the cream cheese mixture.
4. Roll the tortillas tightly into wraps.

Nutritional Value:

- Calories: Approximately 400 per wrap
- Protein: 20g
- Fat: 25g
- Carbohydrates: 30g

- Fiber: 8g

Cooking Time: 15 minutes.

1.Greek Salad with Grilled Chicken

Ingredients

- 1 pound (450g) boneless, skinless chicken breasts
- 1 teaspoon dried oregano
- teaspoon dried thyme
- Salt and pepper to taste
- tablespoons olive oil (divided)
- 4 cups (about 200g) mixed salad greens (lettuce, spinach, arugula, etc.)
- 1 cucumber, sliced
- 1 cup (150g) cherry tomatoes, halved
- 1 red onion, thinly sliced
- cup (150g) feta cheese, crumbled 1/2 cup (75g) Kalamata olives, pitted

For the Dressing:

- 1/4 cup (60ml) extra virgin olive oil
- tablespoons red wine vinegar
- 1 teaspoon Dijon mustard
- 1 clove garlic, minced Salt and pepper to taste

Preparation:

Marinate the Chicken:

1. In a bowl, mix the chicken breasts with oregano, thyme, salt, pepper, and 1 tablespoon of olive oil. Marinate for at least 30 minutes. Grill the Chicken:

2. Heat the grill or grill pan to medium-high.

3. Grill the marinated chicken for about 6-8 minutes per side or until cooked through.

4. Let the chicken rest for a few minutes before slicing.

Prepare the Salad:

- In a large bowl, combine salad greens, cucumber, cherry tomatoes, red onion, feta cheese, and Kalamata olives.

Make the Dressing:

- Whisk together the extra virgin olive oil, red wine vinegar, Dijon mustard, minced garlic, salt, and pepper in a small bowl.

Prepare the Salad:

- Place the grilled chicken slices on top of the salad. Dress the salad and chicken with the dressing.

Nutritional Value:

- This salad provides a balanced mix of protein, healthy fats, and a variety of vitamins and minerals.
- Chicken: High in protein, low in fat.
- Olive oil and feta cheese: Good sources of healthy fats.
- Vegetables: Rich in vitamins and minerals.

Cooking Time:

Marinating time: 30 minutes

Grilling time: 12-16 minutes

Enjoy your delicious and nutritious Greek Salad with Grilled Chicken!

Ingredients

- cup quinoa

- cups water

- 1 tablespoon olive oil

- 1 clove garlic, minced

- 1 cup cherry tomatoes, halved

- 1 cucumber, diced

- 1/2 red onion, finely chopped

- 1/4 cup Kalamata olives, sliced

- 1/4 cup feta cheese, crumbled

- 1/4 cup fresh parsley, chopped

- Salt and pepper to taste

- Lemon wedges for serving

Nutritional Value (per serving):

- Calories: Approximately 400

- Protein: 12g

- Fat: 16g

- Carbohydrates: 55g

- Fiber: 8g

Preparation:

1. Rinse the quinoa with cool water. Combine quinoa and water in a saucepan. Bring to a boil, then lower to a low heat, cover, and leave for 15 minutes, or until the water has been absorbed.

2. Using a fork, fluff the rice.

3. Warm the olive oil in a large skillet over medium heat. Sauté the minced garlic for 1-2 minutes, or until fragrant.

4. Add cherry tomatoes, cucumber, and red onion to the skillet. Cook for 3-4 minutes until vegetables are slightly softened.

5. Stir in cooked quinoa, Kalamata olives, and season with salt and pepper. Cook for an additional 2-3 minutes.

6. Remove from heat and transfer the mixture to serving bowls.

7. Top each bowl with crumbled feta, chopped parsley, and a squeeze of lemon juice.

8. Serve immediately and enjoy your nutritious Mediterranean Quinoa Bowl!

Cooking Time: Approximately 20 minutes

3. Lemon Herb Baked Fish

Ingredients:

- 4 fillets of white fish (such as cod or tilapia)
- 2 tablespoons olive oil
- lemon (juiced)
- cloves garlic (minced)

- 1 teaspoon dried oregano

- 1 teaspoon dried thyme

- Salt and pepper to taste Lemon slices for garnish

Preparation:

1. Preheat the oven to 375°F (190°C).

2. Place the fish fillets in a baking dish and season with salt and pepper.

3. In a small bowl, mix together olive oil, lemon juice, minced garlic, oregano, and thyme.

4. Pour the herb mixture over the fish fillets, ensuring they are evenly coated.

5. To enhance flavor, place lemon slices on top of each fillet.

6. Cover the baking dish with aluminum foil and bake for 15-20 minutes, or until the fish flakes easily with a fork.

7. Uncover and broil for an additional 2-3 minutes to lightly brown the top.

8. If preferred, garnish with fresh herbs and serve.

Nutritional Value (per serving):

- Calories: Approximately 200 kcal

- Protein: 25g

- Fat: 10g

- Carbohydrates: 3g

- Fiber: 1g

- Sugars: 1g

- Sodium: 300mg

Cooking Time:

15-20 minutes at 375°F (190°C) plus an additional 2-3 minutes under the broiler.

4. Chickpea and Spinach Stew

Ingredients:

- cup dried chickpeas, soaked overnight

- tablespoons olive oil

- 1 onion, finely chopped

- 3 cloves garlic, minced

- 1 teaspoon ground cumin

- 1 teaspoon ground coriander

- 1/2 teaspoon smoked paprika

- 1/4 teaspoon cayenne pepper (optional for heat)

- 1 can (14 oz) diced tomatoes

- cups vegetable broth

- cups fresh spinach, chopped Salt and pepper to taste

Preparation:

1. Rinse soaked chickpeas and set aside.

2. Warm the olive oil in a big pot over medium heat. Cook until the onion has softened.

3. Add minced garlic, cumin, coriander, paprika, and cayenne. Cook for 1-2 minutes until fragrant. Stir in soaked chickpeas, diced tomatoes (with juice), and vegetable broth. Bring to a boil, then reduce heat and simmer for 1.5 to 2 hours or until chickpeas are tender.

4. Add chopped spinach and cook for an additional 5-10 minutes until wilted.

5. Season with salt and pepper to taste.

Nutritional Value (per serving):

- Calories: Approximately 300
- Protein: 15g
- Fiber: 10g

- Fat: 10g

- Carbohydrates: 40g

Cooking Time:

Approximately 2 hours and 15 minutes.

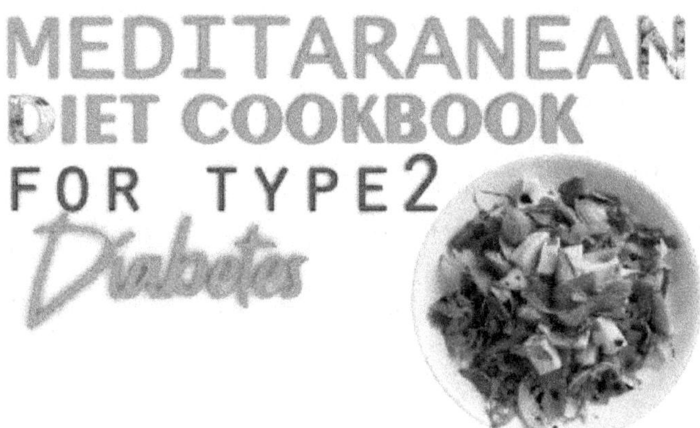

5. Eggplant Parmesan

Ingredients

- 2 large eggplants, sliced into 1/2-inch rounds

- 2 cups breadcrumbs

- 1 cup grated Parmesan cheese

- 3 eggs, beaten

- 2 cups marinara sauce

- 2 cups shredded mozzarella cheese

- 1/4 cup chopped fresh basil

- Salt and pepper to taste Olive oil for frying

Preparation:

1. Preheat oven to 375°F (190°C).

2. Sprinkle eggplant slices with salt, let sit for 30 minutes, then rinse and pat dry.

3. In one bowl, combine breadcrumbs and grated Parmesan. Dip eggplant slices in beaten eggs, then coat with breadcrumb mixture.

4. In a skillet over medium heat, heat the olive oil. Fry eggplant slices for 2-3 minutes per side, or until golden brown. Dry with paper towels.

5. Spread a thin layer of marinara sauce in a baking dish. Arrange a layer of fried eggplant slices on top, followed by a layer of mozzarella, and repeat until all ingredients have been utilized, finishing with a layer of sauce and mozzarella on top.

6. 25-30 minutes, or until the cheese is bubbling and golden.

7. Garnish with chopped basil before serving.

Nutritional Value (per serving):

- Calories: 400
- Protein: 18g
- Carbohydrates: 35g
- Fat: 20g

- Fiber: 7g

- Sugar: 10g

Cooking Time: 1 hour (including preparation and baking).

6. Mediterranean Veggie Wrap

Ingredients:

- 1 whole-grain wrap

- 1/2 cup cherry tomatoes, sliced

- 1/2 cucumber, thinly sliced

- 1/4 cup red onion, finely chopped

- 1/4 cup Kalamata olives, pitted and sliced

- 1/4 cup feta cheese, crumbled

- 1/2 cup mixed greens (spinach, arugula, or lettuce)

- 1 tablespoon extra virgin olive oil

- 1 teaspoon balsamic vinegar

- 1/2 teaspoon dried oregano Salt and pepper to taste

Preparation:

1. In a bowl, combine cherry tomatoes, cucumber, red onion, olives, feta cheese, and mixed greens.

2. Drizzle olive oil and balsamic vinegar over the veggies. Sprinkle with dried oregano, salt, and pepper. Toss until well-coated.

3. Spread the whole-grain wrap out on a flat surface.

4. Spoon the prepared veggie mixture onto the center of the wrap.

5. Fold in the sides of the wrap and then roll it up tightly.

6. Optionally, secure the wrap with a toothpick or wrap it in parchment paper for easier handling.

Nutritional Value (Approximate):

- Calories: 400 kcal

- Protein: 12g

- Carbohydrates: 35g

- Fiber: 8g

- Fat: 25g

- Saturated Fat: 7g

- Cholesterol: 25mg

- Sodium: 600mg

Cooking Time:

Preparation time: 15 minutes

7. Roasted Red Pepper and Walnut Dip

Ingredients:

- 2 large red bell peppers

- 1 cup walnuts, toasted

- 3 cloves garlic

- 2 tablespoons olive oil

- 1 tablespoon lemon juice

- 1 teaspoon ground cumin

- Salt and pepper to taste

- Optional: 1/4 teaspoon cayenne pepper for added heat

Preparation:

1. Preheat the oven to 400°F (200°C).

2. Place the red peppers on a baking sheet and roast for 25-30 minutes, turning occasionally, until the skin is charred and blistered.

3. Remove peppers from the oven, place them in a bowl, and cover with plastic wrap. Let them cool for 15 minutes.

4. Peel the skin off the peppers, remove seeds, and chop into smaller pieces.

5. In a food processor, combine the roasted red peppers, toasted walnuts, garlic, olive oil, lemon juice, cumin, salt, and pepper. Blend until smooth.

6. Taste and adjust seasoning, adding cayenne pepper if desired for extra spiciness. Transfer the dip to a serving bowl, drizzle with olive oil, and garnish with chopped parsley or additional toasted walnuts if desired.

Nutritional Value (per serving):

- Calories: Approximately 150
- Protein: 3g
- Fat: 13g
- Carbohydrates: 6g
- Fiber: 2g
- Sugar: 2g
- Sodium: Varies based on added salt

Cooking Time:

30-35 minutes (roasting peppers)

10 minutes (preparation)

8. Mediterranean Quiche with Spinach and Feta

Ingredients:

- 1 pre-made pie crust
- 1 cup fresh spinach, chopped
- 1/2 cup feta cheese, crumbled
- 1/2 cup cherry tomatoes, halved
- 1/4 cup red onion, finely chopped
- 4 large eggs
- 1 cup whole milk
- 1/2 teaspoon dried oregano Salt and pepper to taste

Preparation:

1. Preheat the oven to 375°F (190°C).

2. Place the pre-made pie crust in a quiche pan or pie dish.

3. In a skillet, sauté the chopped spinach and red onion until softened.

4. In a bowl, whisk together eggs, milk, dried oregano, salt, and pepper.

5. Spread the sautéed spinach and red onion evenly over the pie crust.

6. Sprinkle feta cheese and halved cherry tomatoes on top.

7. Pour the egg mixture over the pie crust filling.

8. Bake for 30-35 minutes, or until the quiche is set and the crust is golden brown, in a preheated oven.

9. Allow the quiche to cool slightly before slicing.

Nutritional Value (per serving):

49

- Calories: Approximately 300

- Protein: 12g

- Fat: 20g

- Carbohydrates: 18g

- Fiber: 2g

9. Grilled Shrimp Skewers

Ingredients:

- pound (450g) big peeled and deveined shrimp

- tablespoons olive oil

- 2 cloves garlic, minced

- 1 teaspoon paprika

- 1 teaspoon dried oregano

- 1/2 teaspoon salt

- 1/4 teaspoon black pepper

- 1 tablespoon lemon juice

- Wooden skewers that have been soaked in water for 30 minutes

Preparation:

1. In a bowl, combine olive oil, minced garlic, paprika, dried oregano, salt, black pepper, and lemon juice to create the marinade.

2. Pat dry the shrimp with paper towels and add them to the marinade. Toss to coat evenly. Allow to marinate for at least 30 minutes in the refrigerator.

3. Preheat the grill to medium-high heat.

4. Thread the moistened wooden skewers with the marinated shrimp.

5. Grill the shrimp skewers for 2-3 minutes per side or until they turn opaque and slightly charred.

6. Serve immediately, garnished with fresh lemon wedges.

Nutritional Value (per serving):

- Calories: Approximately 200 kcal

- Protein: 25g

- Fat: 10g

- Carbohydrates: 2g

- Fiber: 0.5g

- Sugars: 0.5g

- Cholesterol: 180mg

- Sodium: 500mg

Cooking Time:

Marinating Time: 30 minutes

Grilling Time: 4-6 minutes

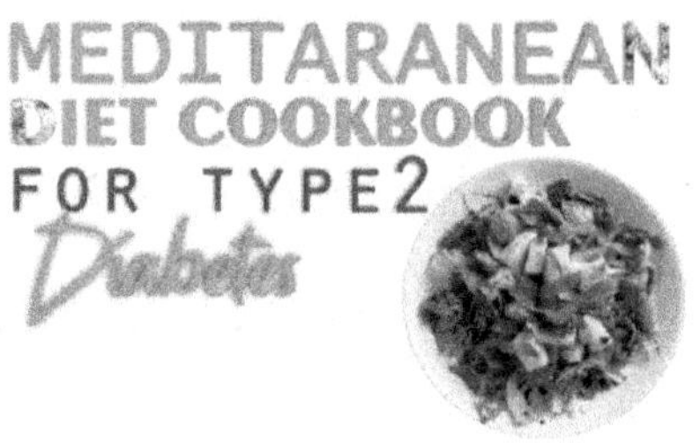

Ingredients:

- 1 cup dried green or brown lentils
- 1 large onion, finely chopped
- 3 cloves garlic, minced
- 2 carrots, diced
- 2 celery stalks, chopped
- 1 can (14 oz) diced tomatoes
- 6 cups vegetable broth
- 2 teaspoons ground cumin
- 1 teaspoon dried oregano
- teaspoon paprika
- Salt and pepper to taste
- tablespoons olive oil Fresh parsley for garnish

Preparation:

1. Set lentils aside after rinsing them under cool water.
2. Warm the olive oil in a big pot over medium heat. Sauté the onions and garlic until softened.
3. Cook for 5 minutes after adding carrots and celery.
4. Cook for an additional 2 minutes after adding cumin, oregano, and paprika.
5. Pour in the veggie broth and season with salt and pepper. Bring the water to a boil.
6. Reduce the heat to low, cover, and cook for 25-30 minutes, or until the lentils are cooked.
7. If necessary, adjust the seasoning.
8. Serve hot, garnished with fresh parsley.

Nutritional Value (per serving):

Calories: 250

Protein: 15g

Carbohydrates: 40g

Fiber: 15g

Fat: 5g Cooking Time:

Approximately 35 minutes

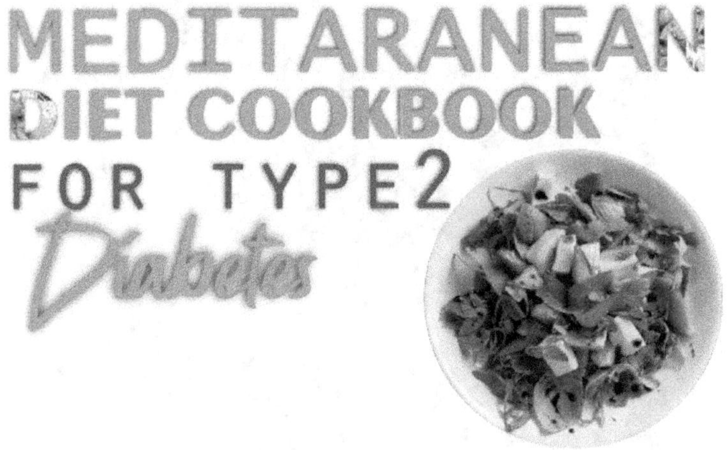

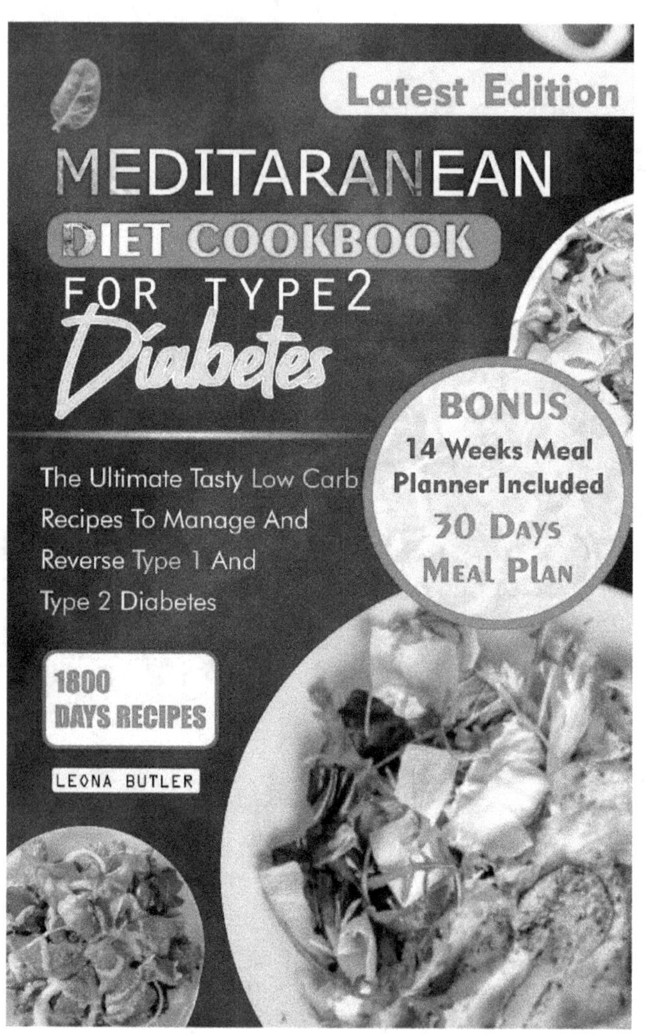

Latest Edition
MEDITARANEAN
DIET COOKBOOK
FOR TYPE2
Diabetes
The Ultimate Tasty Low Carb
Recipes To Manage And
Reverse Type 1 And
Type 2 Diabetes
BONUS
14 Weeks Meal
Planner Included
30 Days
Meal Plan
1800
DAYS RECIPES
LEONA BUTLER

1. Grilled Lemon Herb Chicken with Roasted Vegetables

Ingredients:

- 4 boneless, skinless chicken breasts
- lemons (juiced and zested)
- tablespoons olive oil
- 2 cloves garlic (minced)
- 1 teaspoon dried oregano
- 1 teaspoon dried thyme
- Salt and pepper to taste
- pound baby potatoes (halved)
- cups baby carrots
- 1 red bell pepper (sliced)
- 1 yellow bell pepper (sliced)
- 1 zucchini (sliced)
- Fresh parsley for garnish

Nutritional Value (per serving):

- Calories: 400

- Protein: 30g

- Carbohydrates: 25g

- Fat: 20g

- Fiber: 5g

Preparation:

1. In a bowl, combine lemon juice, lemon zest, olive oil, minced garlic, dried oregano, dried thyme, salt, and pepper to create the marinade.

2. Place chicken breasts in a resealable plastic bag, pour half of the marinade over them, and refrigerate for at least 30 minutes.

3. Preheat the grill to medium-high heat.

4. In a separate bowl, toss halved baby potatoes, baby carrots, sliced bell peppers, and zucchini with the remaining marinade.

5. Thread marinated chicken onto skewers.

6. Grill chicken skewers for 6-8 minutes per side or until fully cooked.

7. At the same time, spread the marinated vegetables on a baking sheet and roast in the oven at 400°F (200°C) for 20-25 minutes or until tender.

8. Garnish the grilled chicken with fresh parsley before serving.

Cooking Time:

Grilling Chicken: 12-16 minutes

Roasting Vegetables: 20-25 minutes

2. Baked Salmon with Mediterranean Quinoa Salad

Ingredients:

- For Baked Salmon:

- 4 salmon fillets (about 6 oz each)

- 2 tablespoons olive oil

- teaspoon lemon juice

- cloves garlic, minced

- Salt and pepper to taste

- For Mediterranean Quinoa Salad:

- cup quinoa

- cups water

- 1 cup cherry tomatoes, halved

- 1 cucumber, diced

- 1/2 red onion, finely chopped

- 1/4 cup Kalamata olives, sliced

- 1/4 cup feta cheese, crumbled 2 tablespoons fresh parsley, chopped

Preparation:

For Baked Salmon:

1. Preheat the oven to 400°F (200°C).

2. In a small bowl, mix olive oil, lemon juice, minced garlic, salt, and pepper.

3. Line a baking sheet with parchment paper and place the salmon fillets on it.

4. Brush the salmon fillets with the olive oil mixture.

5. Bake for 12-15 minutes or until the salmon flakes easily with a fork. For Mediterranean Quinoa Salad:

6. Rinse quinoa under cold water.

7. In a saucepan, combine quinoa and water.

8. Bring to a boil, then lower to a low heat, cover, and leave for 15 minutes, or until the water has been absorbed.

9. Allow quinoa to cool before fluffing with a fork.

10. In a large bowl, combine cooked quinoa, cherry tomatoes, cucumber, red onion, Kalamata olives, feta cheese, and parsley.

11. Drizzle with olive oil and toss gently to combine.

12. Season with salt and pepper to taste.

Nutritional Value:

- Baked Salmon: Each 6 oz fillet provides approximately 350 calories, 22g of protein, and rich in omega-3 fatty acids.

- Mediterranean Quinoa Salad: A serving offers around 250 calories, 8g of protein, and a variety of vitamins and minerals.

Cooking Time:

Baked Salmon: 12-15 minutes at 400°F (200°C).

Mediterranean Quinoa Salad: About 20 minutes for quinoa preparation, plus additional time for cooling and assembling the salad.

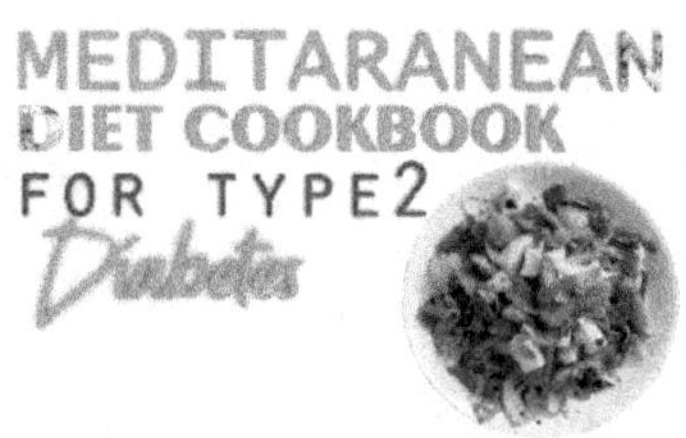

3. Chickpea and Spinach Stew with Whole Grain Couscous

Ingredients:

- cup dried chickpeas, soaked overnight
- tbsp olive oil
- 1 onion, finely chopped
- 3 cloves garlic, minced
- 1 tsp cumin powder
- 1 tsp coriander powder
- 1/2 tsp paprika
- 1 can (14 oz) diced tomatoes
- 4 cups fresh spinach, chopped
- 4 cups vegetable broth Salt and pepper to taste

For Whole Grain Couscous:

- 1 cup whole grain couscous
- 1 1/2 cups water
- 1 tbsp olive oil

- Salt to taste

Preparation:

1. Warm the olive oil in a big pot over medium heat. Cook until the onions are transparent.

2. Add minced garlic, cumin powder, coriander powder, and paprika. Cook for 2 minutes until fragrant.

3. Drain soaked chickpeas and add them to the pot. Stir well.

4. Pour in diced tomatoes, vegetable broth, salt, and pepper. Bring to a boil, then reduce heat and simmer for 45-60 minutes or until chickpeas are tender.

5. In a separate pot, bring water, olive oil, and salt to a boil. Add whole grain couscous, cover, and let it simmer for 10 minutes or until water is absorbed. Fluff with a fork.

6. Add chopped spinach to the chickpea stew and cook until wilted.

7. Serve the chickpea and spinach stew over the whole grain couscous.

Nutritional Value (per serving):

- Calories: ~400

- Protein: ~15g Fiber: ~12g

- Healthy fats: ~10g

- Carbohydrates: ~60g

Cooking Time:

Chickpea stew: 45-60 minutes

Whole grain couscous: 10 minutes

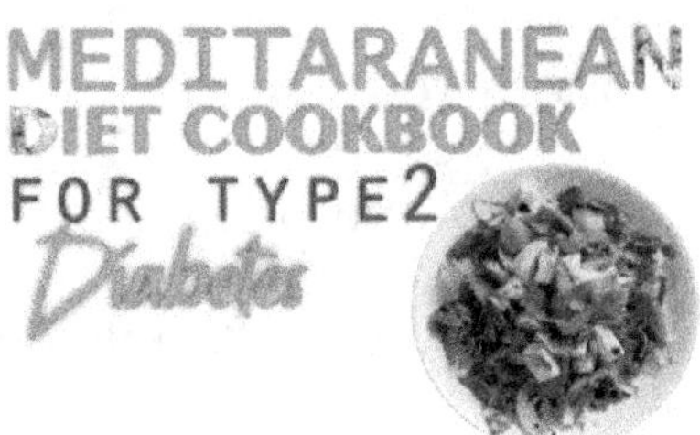

4. Greek Salad with Grilled Shrimp

Ingredients:

- pound (450g) big peeled and deveined shrimp

- tablespoons olive oil

- 1 teaspoon dried oregano Salt and pepper to taste

For the Greek Salad:

- 4 cups (about 500g) mixed salad greens

- 1 cup cherry tomatoes, halved

- 1 cucumber, diced

- 1 red onion, thinly sliced

- cup Kalamata olives, pitted 1 cup feta cheese, crumbled

For the Dressing:

- 1/4 cup (60ml) extra-virgin olive oil

- tablespoons red wine vinegar

- 1 teaspoon Dijon mustard

- 1 clove garlic, minced Salt and pepper to taste

Preparation:

- In a bowl, marinate the shrimp with olive oil, oregano, salt, and pepper. Let it sit for 15 minutes.
- Heat the grill or grill pan to medium-high.
- Grill the shrimp for 2-3 minutes per side or until cooked through.
- In a large salad bowl, combine the salad greens, cherry tomatoes, cucumber, red onion, olives, and feta cheese.
- In a small bowl, whisk together the olive oil, red wine vinegar, Dijon mustard, garlic, salt, and pepper to create the dressing.
- Toss the salad with the dressing to mix it.
- Top the salad with grilled shrimp.
- Serve immediately.

Nutritional Value:

- Calories: Approximately 400 calories per serving.

- Protein: 25g

- Fat: 30g

- Carbohydrates: 15g

- Fiber: 5g

Cooking Time:

Grilling shrimp: 6-8 minutes

Assembling salad: 10 minutes

5. Eggplant Parmesan with Tomato Basil Sauce

Ingredients:

- 2 large eggplants, sliced into 1/2-inch rounds

- 2 cups breadcrumbs

- 1 cup grated Parmesan cheese

- 4 eggs, beaten

- 3 cups marinara sauce

- cup fresh basil, chopped

- cups shredded mozzarella cheese

- Salt and pepper to taste

- Olive oil for frying

Nutritional Value (per serving):

- Calories: Approximately 450

- Protein: 18g

- Carbohydrates: 35g

- Fat: 25g

- Fiber: 7g

Preparation:

1. Preheat the oven to 375°F (190°C).

2. Season eggplant slices with salt and let them sit for 15 minutes to draw out excess moisture.

3. In a shallow dish, combine breadcrumbs and grated Parmesan.

4. Dip each eggplant slice in beaten eggs, then coat with breadcrumb mixture.

5. Heat olive oil in a pan over medium heat, and fry eggplant slices until golden brown.

6. In a separate bowl, mix marinara sauce and fresh basil.

7. In a baking dish, layer fried eggplant slices, marinara sauce, and shredded mozzarella.

8. Repeat the layers, finishing with a layer of mozzarella on top.

9. Bake for 25-30 minutes, or until the cheese is bubbling and golden, in a preheated oven.

10. Allow for a few minutes of cooling before serving.

Enjoy your delicious Eggplant Parmesan with Tomato Basil Sauce!

Ingredients:

- 1 cup dry lentils
- 4 cups vegetable broth
- onion, diced
- carrots, sliced
- celery stalks, chopped
- cloves garlic, minced
- 1 can (14 oz) diced tomatoes
- 1 teaspoon dried thyme
- 1 teaspoon ground cumin
- 1/2 teaspoon smoked paprika
- Salt and pepper to taste
- 4 cups water
- 2 cups mixed vegetables (e.g., broccoli, zucchini)
- cup spinach, chopped

For the Whole Wheat Bread:

- cups whole wheat flour

- cup all-purpose flour

- 1 tablespoon sugar

- 1 teaspoon salt

- 1 tablespoon active dry yeast

- 1 cup warm water 2 tablespoons olive oil

Preparation:

1. In a large pot, add lentils and vegetable broth. Bring to a boil, then reduce to a low heat and cook for 20 minutes.

2. In a separate pan, soften the onion, carrots, celery, and garlic. Combine this mixture with the lentils.

3. Add diced tomatoes, thyme, cumin, smoked paprika, salt, and pepper to taste. Cook for another 15 minutes.

4. Pour in the water and stir in the vegetables. Simmer for 15-20 minutes, or until all vegetables are soft.

5. Add chopped spinach and cook until wilted.

6. For the Whole Wheat Bread, combine flours, sugar, and salt in a bowl. Dissolve yeast in warm water, then add to the flour mixture along with olive oil. Knead until smooth, let rise for 1 hour, then shape into a loaf and bake at 375°F (190°C) for 25-30 minutes.

Nutritional Value (per serving):

- Calories: 400

- Protein: 18g

- Carbohydrates: 72g

- Fiber: 15g

- Fat: 7g Sodium: 800mg

Cooking Time:

Lentil and Vegetable Soup: approximately 1 hour

Whole Wheat Bread: approximately 2 hours (including rising time and baking)

7. Quinoa-Stuffed Bell Peppers with Feta Cheese

Ingredients:

- 4 large bell peppers
- cup quinoa
- cups vegetable broth
- 1 can (15 oz) black beans, drained and rinsed
- cup corn kernels (fresh or frozen)
- 1 cup diced tomatoes
- cup diced red onion
- cloves garlic, minced
- 1 teaspoon cumin
- 1 teaspoon chili powder

- Salt and pepper to taste

- 1 cup crumbled feta cheese Fresh cilantro for garnish

Preparation:

1. Preheat the oven to 375°F (190°C).

2. Remove the tops of the bell peppers and discard the seeds and membranes.

3. In a medium saucepan, combine quinoa and vegetable broth. Bring to a boil, then reduce heat, cover, and simmer for 15-20 minutes until quinoa is cooked and liquid is absorbed.

4. In a large bowl, mix cooked quinoa, black beans, corn, tomatoes, red onion, garlic, cumin, chili powder, salt, and pepper.

5. Stuff each bell pepper with the quinoa mixture and place in a baking dish.

6. Top each stuffed pepper with crumbled feta cheese.

7. Bake the baking dish for 25-30 minutes, covered with foil.

8. Remove the foil and continue baking for 10 minutes, or until the cheese is melted and bubbling.

9. Garnish with fresh cilantro before serving.

Nutritional Value (per serving):

- Calories: ~350

- Protein: ~15g

- Carbohydrates: ~50g

- Fat: ~10g

- Fiber: ~8g

Cooking Time:

Approximately 45-50 minutes.

8. Lemon Garlic Roasted Chicken with Mediterranean Veggie Skewers

Ingredients:

For Lemon Garlic Roasted Chicken:

- whole chicken (about 3-4 pounds)

- 4 cloves garlic, minced

- lemon, juiced and zested

- tablespoons olive oil

- teaspoon dried oregano

- Salt and pepper to taste

For Mediterranean Veggie Skewers:

- zucchinis, sliced into rounds

- 1 bell pepper, cut into chunks

- 1 red onion, cut into wedges

- cup cherry tomatoes

- tablespoons olive oil

- 1 teaspoon dried thyme Salt and pepper to taste

Preparation:

Preheat the oven to 400°F (200°C).

Lemon Garlic Roasted Chicken:

1. Rinse the chicken and blot it dry with paper towels.

2. In a small bowl, mix minced garlic, lemon juice, lemon zest, olive oil, dried oregano, salt, and pepper to create a marinade.

3. Rub the chicken inside and out with the marinade, ensuring an even coating.

4. Place the chicken in a roasting pan and roast in the preheated oven for approximately 1 hour and 15 minutes or until the internal temperature reaches 165°F (74°C).

Mediterranean Veggie Skewers:

1. In a bowl, toss zucchini rounds, bell pepper chunks, red onion wedges, and cherry tomatoes with olive oil, dried thyme, salt, and pepper.

78

2. Thread the seasoned vegetables onto skewers alternately.

3. Place the skewers on a baking sheet and roast in the oven for about 20-25 minutes or until the veggies are tender.

Cooking Time:

- Lemon Garlic Roasted Chicken: Approximately 1 hour and 15 minutes.

- Mediterranean Veggie Skewers: Approximately 20-25 minutes.

Enjoy your flavorful Lemon Garlic Roasted Chicken with Mediterranean Veggie Skewers!

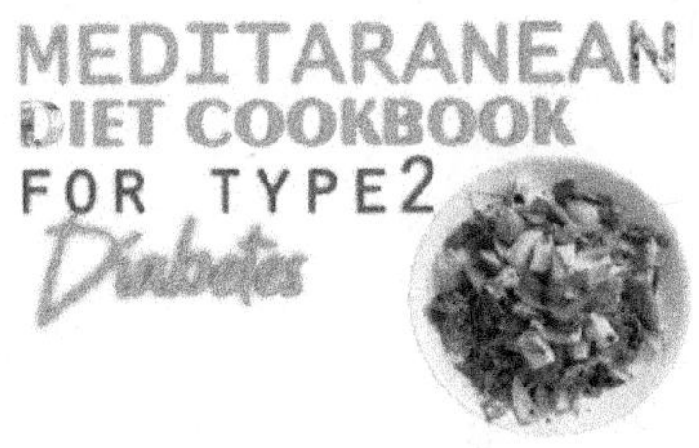

9. Baked Cod with Olive and Tomato Relish

Ingredients:

- 4 cod fillets (about 6 ounces each)
- cup cherry tomatoes, halved
- 1/2 cup Kalamata olives, sliced
- tablespoons extra-virgin olive oil
- 2 tablespoons fresh parsley, chopped
- 2 cloves garlic, minced
- 1 teaspoon dried oregano
- Salt and pepper to taste
- Lemon wedges for serving

For Nutritional Value (per serving):

- Calories: Approximately 300
- Protein: 30g
- Fat: 15g
- Carbohydrates: 6g
- Fiber: 2g

Preparation:

1. Preheat the oven to 400°F (200°C).

2. Place the fish fillets on a baking dish after patting them dry.

3. In a bowl, combine cherry tomatoes, Kalamata olives, olive oil, parsley, garlic, oregano, salt, and pepper. Mix well.

4. Spoon the olive and tomato relish over the cod fillets, ensuring even distribution.

5. Cover the baking dish with foil and bake for 15-20 minutes or until the cod is opaque and flakes easily with a fork.

6. Remove the foil during the last 5 minutes to allow the top to brown slightly. Serve the baked cod with lemon wedges for a refreshing touch.

7. Enjoy your delicious and nutritious baked cod with olive and tomato relish!

10. Zucchini Noodles with Pesto and Cherry Tomatoes

Ingredients:

- 4 medium-sized zucchini, spiralized

- cup cherry tomatoes, halved

- 1/2 cup fresh basil leaves

- 1/3 cup grated Parmesan cheese

- 1/4 cup pine nuts

- cloves garlic

- 1/2 cup extra-virgin olive oil Salt and pepper to taste

Preparation:

Pesto Sauce:

1. Combine basil, Parmesan, pine nuts, and garlic in a food processor.

2. Pulse until finely chopped.

3. With the processor running, slowly add olive oil until the mixture is smooth.

4. Season with salt and pepper to taste.

Zucchini Noodles:

1. Spiralize the zucchini into noodle-like strands using a spiralizer.
2. Heat a drizzle of olive oil in a big pan over medium heat.
3. Sauté the zucchini noodles for 2-3 minutes until just tender.
4. Season with salt and pepper.

Assembly:

- Toss the zucchini noodles in the pesto sauce until they are well coated.
- Gently fold in the cherry tomatoes.

Serve:

- Divide the zucchini noodle mixture into plates.
- Optionally, sprinkle additional Parmesan and pine nuts on top.

Nutritional Value:

- Calories: Approximately 300 per serving
- Protein: 8g
- Fat: 25g
- Carbohydrates: 10g
- Fiber: 3g
- Sugar: 5g

Cooking Time:

Approximately 15 minutes

Enjoy your healthy and delicious zucchini noodles with pesto and cherry tomatoes!

1. Mediterranean Veggie Skewers

Ingredients:

- 1 large eggplant, cut into 1-inch cubes
- 1 zucchini, sliced into rounds
- 1 red bell pepper, cut into chunks
- 1 yellow bell pepper, cut into chunks
- red onion, peeled and quartered
- Cherry tomatoes
- 1/4 cup olive oil
- tablespoons balsamic vinegar
- 2 cloves garlic, minced
- 1 teaspoon dried oregano
- Salt and pepper to taste Wooden skewers, soaked in water

Preparation:

1. To make the marinade, whisk together olive oil, balsamic vinegar, minced garlic, dried oregano, salt, and pepper in a mixing bowl.

2. In a large mixing basin, combine the eggplant, zucchini, bell peppers, red onion, and cherry tomatoes. Toss the vegetables in the marinade until uniformly coated. Allow at least 30 minutes for it to marinade.

3. Heat the grill or grill pan to medium-high.

4. Thread the marinated vegetables onto the soaked wooden skewers, alternating between different veggies.

5. Grill the skewers for about 10-15 minutes, turning occasionally, until the vegetables are tender and slightly charred.

6. Serve the Mediterranean Veggie Skewers hot, optionally drizzling with extra balsamic vinegar and garnishing with fresh herbs.

Nutritional Value (per serving):

- Calories: Approximately 200 kcal

- Protein: 4g

- Carbohydrates: 20g

- Fiber: 7g

- Fat: 13g

- Vitamin C: 120% DV

- Vitamin A: 25% DV

Cooking Time:

Marinating time: 30 minutes

Grill time: 10-15 minutes

2. Hummus with Veggies

Ingredients:

- can (15 oz) chickpeas, drained and rinsed

- 1/4 cup tahini

- tablespoons extra-virgin olive oil

- 2 cloves garlic, minced

- teaspoon ground cumin
- 1/2 teaspoon salt (adjust to taste)
- tablespoons fresh lemon juice
- 2-4 tablespoons water (adjust for desired consistency)

For Serving:

Assorted fresh veggies (carrots, cucumber, bell peppers)

Preparation:

1. In a food processor, combine chickpeas, tahini, olive oil, garlic, cumin, salt, and lemon juice.
2. Blend until smooth, adding water gradually until desired consistency is reached.
3. Taste and adjust salt or lemon juice as needed.

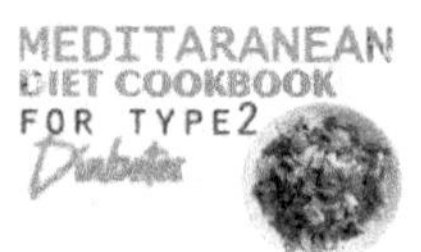

Nutritional Value (per serving):

- Calories: 150
- Protein: 5g
- Fat: 10g
- Carbohydrates: 13g
- Fiber: 3g

Cooking Time:

Preparation: 10 minutes

Total Time: 15 minutes

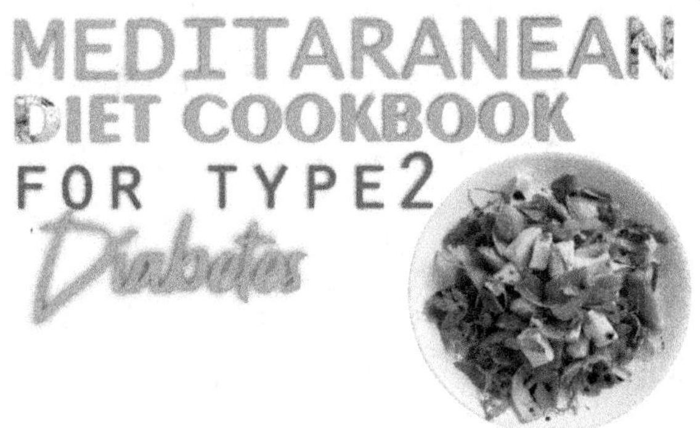

3. Roasted Red Pepper Tapenade

Ingredients:

- 2 large red bell peppers

- 1/2 cup black olives, pitted

- 2 cloves garlic, minced

- 2 tablespoons capers, drained

- 1/4 cup fresh parsley, chopped

- 1/3 cup extra-virgin olive oil Salt and pepper to taste

Preparation:

Roasting Red Peppers:

1. Preheat oven to 450°F (230°C).

2. Place whole red peppers on a baking sheet and roast for 25-30 minutes or until the skin is charred.

3.   Transfer the roasted peppers to a bowl, cover with plastic wrap, and let them cool. Peel, remove seeds, and chop.

Tapenade Assembly:

1. In a food processor, combine roasted red peppers, black olives, minced garlic, capers, and chopped parsley.
2. Pulse until ingredients are finely chopped.
3. While the food processor is running, slowly drip in the olive oil until the mixture is smooth.
4. Season with salt and pepper to taste.

Nutritional Value (per serving):

- Calories: 120
- Fat: 10g
- Carbohydrates: 5g
- Protein: 1g
- Fiber: 2g

Cooking Time:

Roasting peppers: 25-30 minutes

Tapenade assembly: 10 minutes

Serve the Roasted Red Pepper Tapenade with crusty bread or use it as a flavorful spread or topping for various dishes

4. Mediterranean Quinoa Salad

Ingredients:

- cup quinoa
- cups water
- 1 cucumber, diced
- cup cherry tomatoes, halved
- 1/2 cup Kalamata olives, sliced
- 1/4 cup red onion, finely chopped
- 1/4 cup feta cheese, crumbled 1/4 cup fresh parsley, chopped

For the Dressing:

- 1/4 cup extra-virgin olive oil
- tablespoons lemon juice

- 1 clove garlic, minced

- 1 teaspoon dried oregano Salt and pepper to taste

Preparation:

1. Rinse quinoa under cold water. In a saucepan, combine quinoa and water.

2. Bring to a boil, then lower to a low heat, cover, and leave for 15 minutes, or until the water has been absorbed. Allow to cool after fluffing with a fork.

3. In a large bowl, combine cooled quinoa, cucumber, cherry tomatoes, olives, red onion, feta cheese, and parsley.

4. In a small bowl, whisk together olive oil, lemon juice, garlic, oregano, salt, and pepper to create the dressing.

5. Toss the quinoa mixture slightly with the dressing to coat.

6. Allow flavors to mingle for at least 30 minutes before serving.

Nutritional Value (per serving):

- Calories: 320

- Protein: 8g

- Carbohydrates: 34g

- Fiber: 5g

- Fat: 18g

- Saturated Fat: 4g

- Cholesterol: 8mg

- Sodium: 400mg

Cooking Time:

15 minutes for quinoa

30 minutes refrigeration

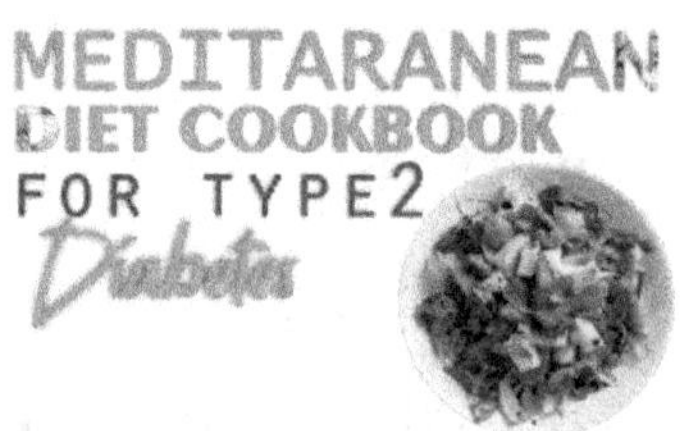

5. Almond and Date Energy Bites

Ingredients:

- 1 cup almonds
- 1 cup pitted dates
- 1/4 cup shredded coconut
- 1 tablespoon chia seeds
- 1/2 teaspoon vanilla extract A pinch of salt

Preparation:

1. In a food processor, combine almonds, dates, shredded coconut, chia seeds, vanilla extract, and a pinch of salt.
2. Blend the mixture until it forms a sticky dough-like consistency.
3. Using your hands, roll little pieces into bite-sized balls.
4. Roll the energy bites in additional shredded coconut to coat if desired.

5. Refrigerate the energy bites for at least 30 minutes on a parchment-lined pan.

Nutritional Value (per serving):

- Calories: Approximately 120

- Protein: 3g

- Fat: 7g

- Carbohydrates: 12g

- Fiber: 2g

- Sugar: 8g

Cooking Time:

Preparation: 15 minutes

Refrigeration: 30 minutes

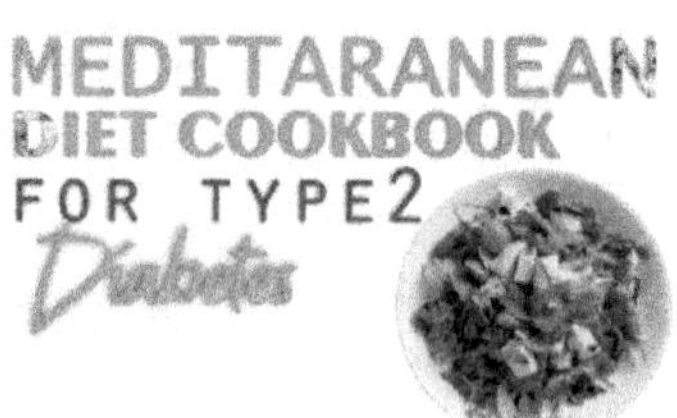

6. Stuffed Grape Leaves

Ingredients:

- 1 cup long-grain white rice 1/2 lb ground lamb or beef
- 1 cup finely chopped onions
- 1/2 cup pine nuts
- 1/4 cup chopped fresh mint
- 1/4 cup chopped fresh dill
- 1/4 cup olive oil
- 1 cup water
- 1/4 cup lemon juice
- Salt and pepper to taste
- 1 jar grape leaves in brine (approx. 60 leaves)

For Cooking:

- lemon, sliced
- cups chicken or vegetable broth

Preparation:

1. Rinse the grape leaves under cold water and soak in warm water to soften.

2. In a pan, sauté onions in olive oil until translucent.

3. Add ground meat and cook until browned.

4. Stir in rice, pine nuts, mint, dill, lemon juice, salt, and pepper.

5. Remove from the heat and set aside to cool.

6. Place a grape leaf flat on a surface, vein side up, and fill with a spoonful of the rice mixture.

7. Fold the sides and roll tightly, forming a compact cylinder.

8. Repeat until all leaves are stuffed.

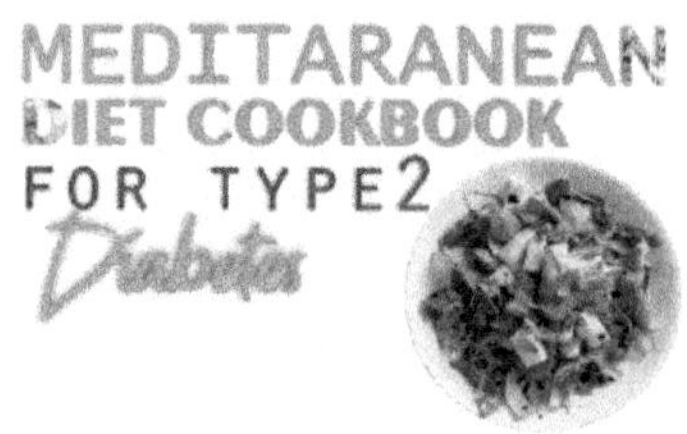

Cooking:

- Line the bottom of a pot with lemon slices.
- Arrange stuffed grape leaves in layers, seam side down.
- Pour chicken or vegetable broth over the top.
- Cook for 45-60 minutes, covered, on low heat.

Nutritional Value (per serving):

- Calories: 250
- Protein: 8g
- Carbohydrates: 30g
- Fat: 12g
- Fiber: 3g

Note: Cooking time may vary, ensure rice is fully cooked. Adjust salt, pepper, and lemon juice according to taste.

Ingredients:

- 1 can (4.375 oz) of sardines in olive oil, drained
- cup cherry tomatoes, diced
- cloves garlic, minced
- 1/4 cup fresh parsley, chopped
- 1 tablespoon extra-virgin olive oil
- Salt and pepper to taste
- Baguette or bread slices for bruschetta

Preparation:

1. In a bowl, combine drained sardines, diced cherry tomatoes, minced garlic, and chopped parsley.
2. Drizzle extra-virgin olive oil over the mixture and season with salt and pepper to taste. Gently toss until well combined.

3. Toast the baguette or bread slices in an oven or toaster until golden brown.

4. Spoon the sardine and tomato mixture onto the toasted bread slices.

5. Serve immediately and enjoy your sardine and tomato bruschetta!

Nutritional Value:

This recipe serves approximately 4 people.

Each serving contains about 250 calories, 15g of protein, 12g of fat, and 20g of carbohydrates.

Cooking Time:

Preparation time: 15 minutes

Cooking time: 5 minutes (toasting the bread)

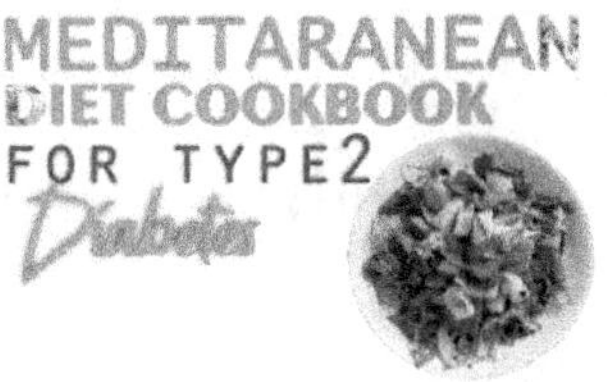

8. Minty Melon Salad

Ingredients:

- 4 cups watermelon, cubed
- 2 cups honeydew melon, diced
- 2 cups cantaloupe, sliced
- 1/4 cup fresh mint leaves, chopped
- tablespoon honey
- tablespoons lime juice
- Optional: Feta cheese crumbles for garnish

Preparation:

1. In a large bowl, combine watermelon, honeydew melon, and cantaloupe.
2. In a small mixing dish, combine honey and lime juice.
3. Pour the honey-lime dressing over the melon mixture and gently toss to coat evenly.

4. Sprinkle fresh mint leaves over the salad and toss again to distribute evenly.

5. Optional: Garnish with feta cheese crumbles for an extra flavor dimension.

6. Serve immediately or refrigerate for a refreshing chilled salad.

Nutritional Value:

- Calories: Approximately 120 per serving (1 cup)
- Fat: 0.5g
- Carbohydrates: 30g
- Fiber: 2g
- Protein: 2g
- Vitamin C: 50% of daily recommended intake

Cooking Time:

Preparation: 15 minutes Optional chilling time: 30 minutes

9. Cucumber and Tzatziki Dip

Ingredients:

- large cucumber, grated

- cups Greek yogurt

- 2 cloves garlic, minced

- 2 tablespoons fresh dill, chopped

- 1 tablespoon olive oil

- 1 tablespoon lemon juice Salt and pepper to taste

Preparation:

1. Squeeze off any extra water after peeling and grating the cucumber.

2. Combine grated cucumber, Greek yogurt, minced garlic, chopped dill, olive oil, and lemon juice in a mixing bowl.

3. Season with salt and pepper to taste after completely mixing. Refrigerate for at least 1 hour to allow flavors to combine.

Nutritional Value:

- Serving size: 2 tablespoons

- Calories: 35

- Protein: 2g

- Fat: 2g

- Carbohydrates: 3g

- Fiber: 0g

- Sugar: 2g

Cooking Time:

Prep time: 15 minutes

Chill time: 1 hour

The Paperback Of This Version Has A Free 14 Weeks Meal Planner

MY WEEKLY MEAL PLANNER

Date

	Breakfast	Lunch	Dinner
MON			
TUE			
WED			
THU			
FRI			
SAT			
SUN			

SHOPPING LIST:

To Do List

NOTES AND TIPS

Day 1:

Breakfast: Mediterranean Veggie Omelette

Lunch: Greek Salad with Grilled Chicken

Dinner: Grilled Lemon Herb Chicken with Roasted Vegetables

Snack: Mediterranean Veggie Skewers

Day 2:

Breakfast: Greek Yogurt Parfait

Lunch: Mediterranean Quinoa Bowl

Dinner: Baked Salmon with Mediterranean Quinoa Salad

Snack: Hummus with Veggies

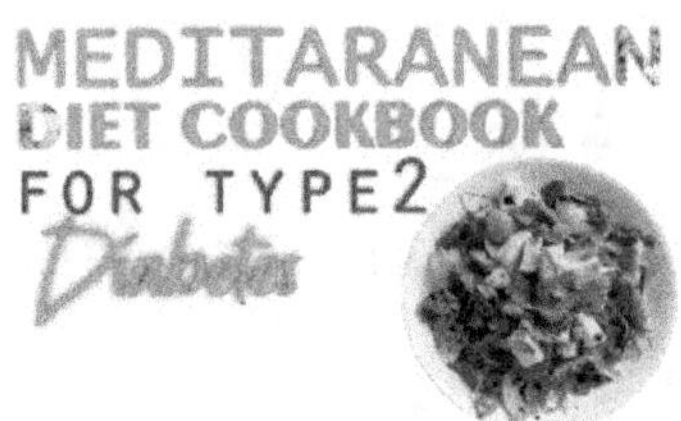

Day 3:

Breakfast: Quinoa Breakfast Bowl

Lunch: Lemon Herb Baked Fish

Dinner: Chickpea and Spinach Stew with Whole Grain Couscous

Snack: Roasted Red Pepper Tapenade

Day 4:

Breakfast: Mediterranean Avocado Toast

Lunch: Chickpea and Spinach Stew

Dinner: Greek Salad with Grilled Shrimp

Snack: Mediterranean Quinoa Salad

Day 5:

Breakfast: Shakshuka

Lunch: Eggplant Parmesan

Dinner: Lentil and Vegetable Soup with a Side of Whole Wheat Bread

Snack: Almond and Date Energy Bites

Day 6:

Breakfast: Mediterranean Chia Pudding

Lunch: Mediterranean Veggie Wrap

Dinner: Quinoa-Stuffed Bell Peppers with Feta Cheese

Snack: Stuffed Grape Leaves

Day 7:

Breakfast: Mediterranean Frittata Muffins

Lunch: Roasted Red Pepper and Walnut Dip

Dinner: Lemon Garlic Roasted Chicken with Mediterranean Veggie Skewers

Snack: Sardine and Tomato Bruschetta

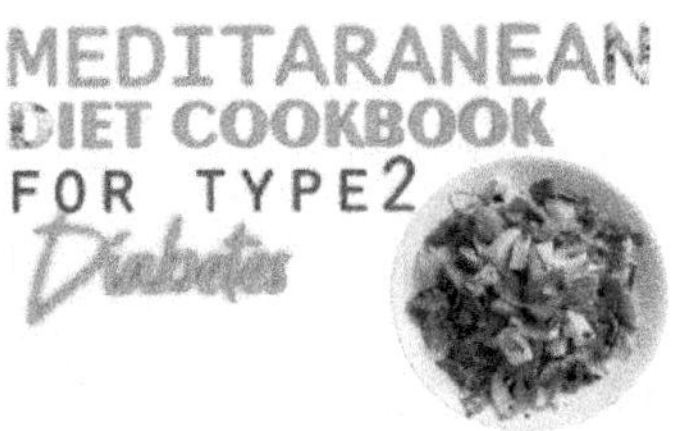

Day 8:

Breakfast: Whole Grain Pancakes with Berries

Lunch: Mediterranean Quiche with Spinach and Feta

Dinner: Baked Cod with Olive and Tomato Relish

Snack: Minty Melon Salad

Day 9:

Breakfast: Mediterranean Breakfast Burrito

Lunch: Grilled Shrimp Skewers

Dinner: Zucchini Noodles with Pesto and Cherry Tomatoes

Snack: Cucumber and Tzatziki Dip

Day 10:

Breakfast: Smoked Salmon and Avocado Wrap

Lunch: Mediterranean Lentil Soup

Dinner: Greek Salad with Grilled Chicken

Snack: Mediterranean Veggie Skewers

Day 11:

Breakfast: Greek Yogurt Parfait

Lunch: Mediterranean Quinoa Bowl

Dinner: Baked Salmon with Mediterranean Quinoa Salad

Snack: Hummus with Veggies

Day 12:

Breakfast: Quinoa Breakfast Bowl

Lunch: Lemon Herb Baked Fish

Dinner: Chickpea and Spinach Stew with Whole Grain Couscous

Snack: Roasted Red Pepper Tapenade

Day 13:

Breakfast: Mediterranean Avocado Toast

Lunch: Chickpea and Spinach Stew

Dinner: Greek Salad with Grilled Shrimp

Snack: Mediterranean Quinoa Salad

Day 14:

Breakfast: Shakshuka

Lunch: Eggplant Parmesan

Dinner: Lentil and Vegetable Soup with a Side of Whole Wheat Bread

Snack: Almond and Date Energy Bites

Day 15:

Breakfast: Mediterranean Chia Pudding

Lunch: Mediterranean Veggie Wrap

Dinner: Quinoa-Stuffed Bell Peppers with Feta Cheese

Snack: Stuffed Grape Leaves

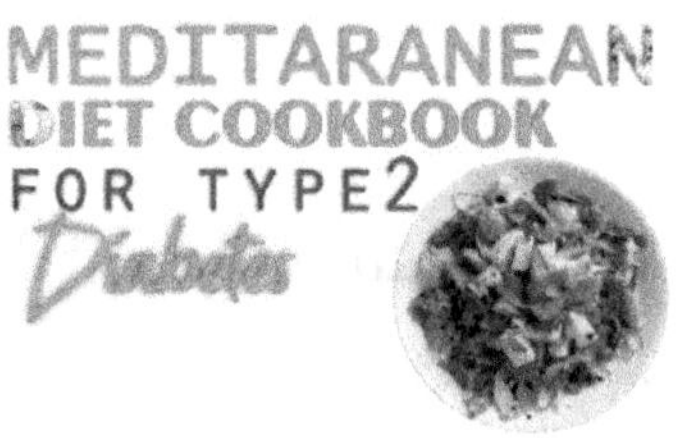

Day 16:

Breakfast: Mediterranean Frittata Muffins

Lunch: Roasted Red Pepper and Walnut Dip

Dinner: Lemon Garlic Roasted Chicken with Mediterranean Veggie Skewers

Snack: Sardine and Tomato Bruschetta

Day 17:

Breakfast: Whole Grain Pancakes with Berries

Lunch: Mediterranean Quiche with Spinach and Feta

Dinner: Baked Cod with Olive and Tomato Relish

Snack: Minty Melon Salad

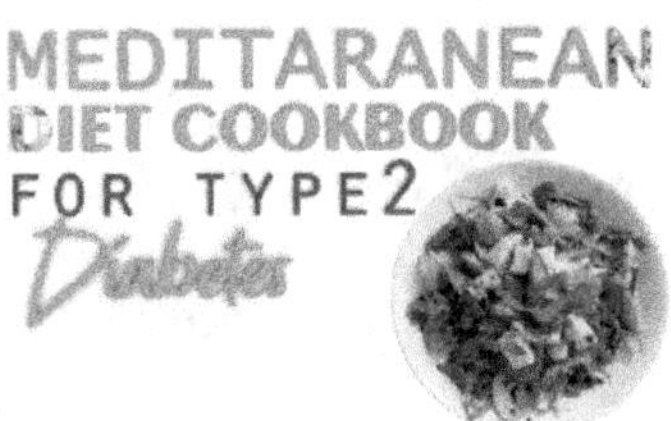

Day 18:

Breakfast: Mediterranean Breakfast Burrito

Lunch: Grilled Shrimp Skewers

Dinner: Zucchini Noodles with Pesto and Cherry Tomatoes

Snack: Cucumber and Tzatziki Dip

Day 19:

Breakfast: Smoked Salmon and Avocado Wrap

Lunch: Mediterranean Lentil Soup

Dinner: Greek Salad with Grilled Chicken

Snack: Mediterranean Veggie Skewers

Day 20:

Breakfast: Greek Yogurt Parfait

Lunch: Mediterranean Quinoa Bowl

Dinner: Baked Salmon with Mediterranean Quinoa Salad

Snack: Hummus with Veggies

Day 21:

Breakfast: Quinoa Breakfast Bowl

Lunch: Lemon Herb Baked Fish

Dinner: Chickpea and Spinach Stew with Whole Grain Couscous

Snack: Roasted Red Pepper Tapenade

Day 22:

Breakfast: Mediterranean Avocado Toast

Lunch: Chickpea and Spinach Stew

Dinner: Greek Salad with Grilled Shrimp

Snack: Mediterranean Quinoa Salad

Day 23:

Breakfast: Shakshuka

Lunch: Eggplant Parmesan

Dinner: Lentil and Vegetable Soup with a Side of Whole Wheat Bread

Snack: Almond and Date Energy Bites

Day 24:

Breakfast: Mediterranean Chia Pudding

Lunch: Mediterranean Veggie Wrap

Dinner: Quinoa-Stuffed Bell Peppers with Feta Cheese

Snack: Stuffed Grape Leaves

Day 25:

Breakfast: Mediterranean Frittata Muffins

Lunch: Roasted Red Pepper and Walnut Dip

Dinner: Lemon Garlic Roasted Chicken with Mediterranean Veggie Skewers

Snack: Sardine and Tomato Bruschetta

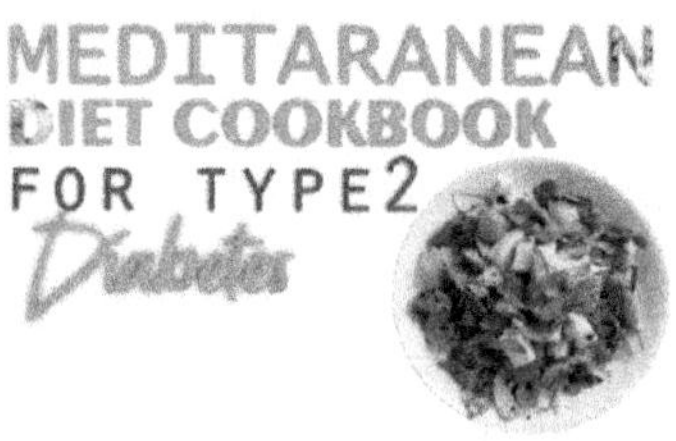

Day 26:

Breakfast: Whole Grain Pancakes with Berries

Lunch: Mediterranean Quiche with Spinach and Feta

Dinner: Baked Cod with Olive and Tomato Relish

Snack: Minty Melon Salad

Day 27:

Breakfast: Mediterranean Breakfast Burrito

Lunch: Grilled Shrimp Skewers

Dinner: Zucchini Noodles with Pesto and Cherry Tomatoes

Snack: Cucumber and Tzatziki Dip

Day 28:

Breakfast: Smoked Salmon and Avocado Wrap

Lunch: Mediterranean Lentil Soup

Dinner: Greek Salad with Grilled Chicken

Snack: Mediterranean Veggie Skewers

Day 29:

Breakfast: Greek Yogurt Parfait

Lunch: Mediterranean Quinoa Bowl

Dinner: Baked Salmon with Mediterranean Quinoa Salad

Snack: Hummus with Veggies

Day 30:

Breakfast: Quinoa Breakfast Bowl

Lunch: Lemon Herb Baked Fish

Dinner: Chickpea and Spinach Stew with Whole Grain Couscous

Snack: Roasted Red Pepper Tapenade

This 30-day meal plan offers a variety of delicious and nutritious Mediterranean-inspired dishes for a well-rounded and satisfying eating experience. Enjoy your meals!

Finally, through a wonderful assortment of nutrient-rich recipes, this Mediterranean diet cookbook offers a flavorful route towards managing type 2 diabetes. Individuals can take proactive actions to improve their overall well-being by embracing the Mediterranean lifestyle's wealth of fresh fruits, vegetables, whole grains, and heart-healthy fats.

This cookbook's expertly created dishes not only cater to taste buds but also match with nutritional requirements for diabetic management. These foods, which are high in antioxidants, fiber, and critical nutrients, help to keep blood sugar levels stable while also supporting cardiovascular health. The use of olive oil, lean meats, and colorful plant-based foods emphasizes the long-term and pleasurable character of this nutritional strategy.

119

As you embark on this gastronomic adventure, keep in mind that following the Mediterranean diet is a holistic commitment to long-term health and energy. Every dish is a modest investment in your well-being, a step toward a healthier, more balanced way of living. You're not just following a diet when you make these choices; you're embracing a lifestyle that prioritizes both the pleasure of eating and the care of your body.

So, make the Mediterranean diet your ally in your quest to a healthy you. Take advantage of this opportunity to relish the delectable flavors, enjoy the delight of nourishing your body, and, ultimately, make a long-term investment in your well-being. Your health is your most valuable asset; preserve it and follow the Mediterranean diet as a guide.

Thank you

Thank you for delving into the Mediterranean Diet Cookbook tailored for managing Type 2 diabetes. Your commitment to exploring these recipes not only fosters a healthier lifestyle but also signifies a proactive step toward holistic well-being. By embracing the rich and nutritious ingredients characteristic of the Mediterranean diet, you are investing in a culinary journey that transcends the mere confines of a cookbook.

This collection aims not only to nourish the body but also to delight the taste buds, making every meal a celebration of health. Your engagement in this culinary experience reflects a dedication to self-care and empowers you with the tools to navigate the challenges of diabetes with flavorful finesse. Your commitment to embracing this lifestyle is not just a

gesture of gratitude but a powerful stride toward

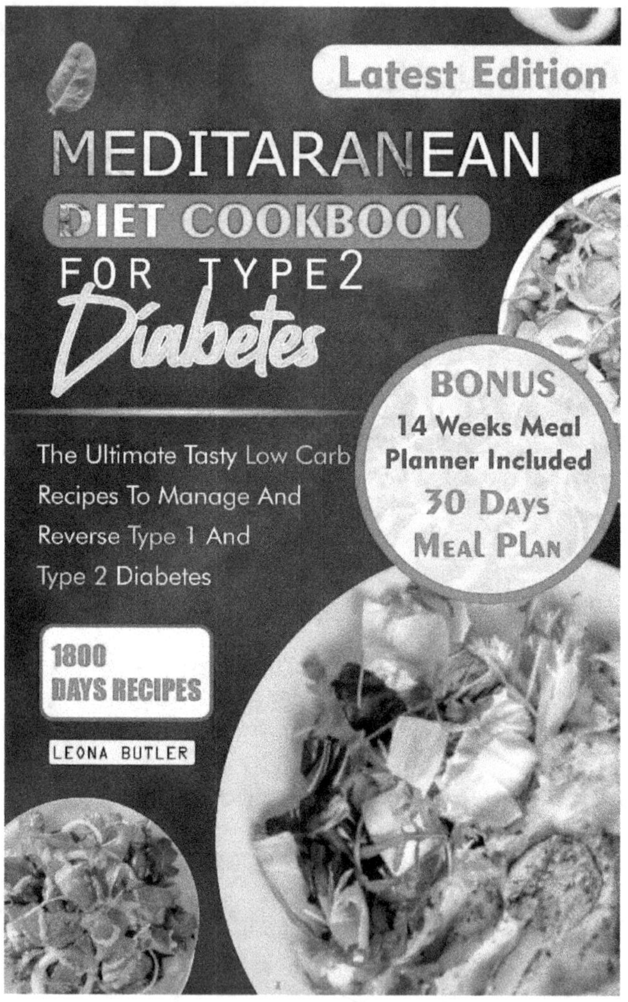

MY WEEKLY MEAL PLANNER

Date

	Breakfast	Lunch	Dinner
MON			
TUE			
WED			
THU			
FRI			
SAT			
SUN			

SHOPPING LIST:

- ·
- ·
- ·
- ·

TO DO LIST

· ·
· ·
· ·
· ·

NOTES
AND TIPS

MY WEEKLY MEAL PLANNER

Date

	Breakfast	Lunch	Dinner
Mon			
Tue			
Wed			
Thu			
Fri			
Sat			
Sun			

SHOPPING LIST:

To Do List

- • . . . .
- • . . . .
- • . . . .
- • . . . .

Notes And Tips

MY WEEKLY MEAL PLANNER

Date

	Breakfast	Lunch	Dinner
MON			
TUE			
WED			
THU			
FRI			
SAT			
SUN			

SHOPPING LIST:

To Do List

- ·························
- ·························
- ·························
- ·························

NOTES
AND TIPS

MY WEEKLY MEAL PLANNER

Date

	Breakfast	Lunch	Dinner
Mon			
Tue			
Wed			
Thu			
Fri			
Sat			
Sun			

SHOPPING LIST:

To Do List

NOTES
AND TIPS

MY WEEKLY MEAL PLANNER

Date

	Breakfast	Lunch	Dinner
MON			
TUE			
WED			
THU			
FRI			
SAT			
SUN			

SHOPPING LIST:

TO DO LIST

- ● -
- ● -
- ● -
- ● -

NOTES
AND TIPS

MY WEEKLY MEAL PLANNER

Date

	Breakfast	Lunch	Dinner
MON			
TUE			
WED			
THU			
FRI			
SAT			
SUN			

SHOPPING LIST:

TO DO LIST

NOTES AND TIPS

MY WEEKLY MEAL PLANNER

Date

	Breakfast	Lunch	Dinner
MON			
TUE			
WED			
THU			
FRI			
SAT			
SUN			

SHOPPING LIST:

TO DO LIST

NOTES AND TIPS

MY WEEKLY MEAL PLANNER

Date

	Breakfast	Lunch	Dinner
MON			
TUE			
WED			
THU			
FRI			
SAT			
SUN			

SHOPPING LIST:

TO DO LIST

NOTES
AND TIPS

MY WEEKLY MEAL PLANNER

Date

	Breakfast	Lunch	Dinner
MON			
TUE			
WED			
THU			
FRI			
SAT			
SUN			

SHOPPING LIST:

To Do List

NOTES
AND TIPS

MY WEEKLY MEAL PLANNER

Date

	Breakfast	Lunch	Dinner
MON			
TUE			
WED			
THU			
FRI			
SAT			
SUN			

SHOPPING LIST:

TO DO LIST

- ● -
- ● -
- ● -
- ● -

NOTES AND TIPS

MY WEEKLY MEAL PLANNER

Date

	Breakfast	Lunch	Dinner
Mon			
Tue			
Wed			
Thu			
Fri			
Sat			
Sun			

SHOPPING LIST:

- ....
- ....
- ....
- ....

To Do List

....
....
....
....

Notes And Tips

MY WEEKLY MEAL PLANNER

Date

	Breakfast	Lunch	Dinner
MON			
TUE			
WED			
THU			
FRI			
SAT			
SUN			

SHOPPING LIST:

TO DO LIST

NOTES AND TIPS

MY WEEKLY MEAL PLANNER

Date

	Breakfast	Lunch	Dinner
MON			
TUE			
WED			
THU			
FRI			
SAT			
SUN			

SHOPPING LIST:

-
-
-
-

TO DO LIST

NOTES
AND TIPS

MY WEEKLY MEAL PLANNER

Date

	Breakfast	Lunch	Dinner
MON			
TUE			
WED			
THU			
FRI			
SAT			
SUN			

SHOPPING LIST:

TO DO LIST

NOTES AND TIPS